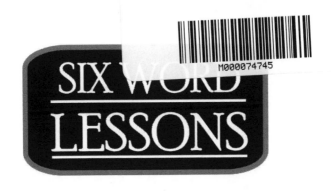

SIX WORD LESSONS

TO BE HEALTHY FOREVER

100 Lessons

to

Achieve and Sustain

Lifelong Health

Deenie Robertson

Activation Health Coaching

ActivationHC.com

Six-Word Lessons to be Healthy Forever – 6wordlessons.com
Editing by Patty Pacelli

Published by Pacelli Publishing
9905 Lake Washington Blvd. NE, #D-103
Bellevue, Washington 98004
Pacellipublishing.com

ISBN- 1-933750-34-0
ISBN- 978-1-933750-34-7

The information in this book comes from years of experience in improving my own nutrition and that of my family's, as well as from my certifications as both a Professional Nutrition Specialist and Nutritional Health Coach.

Over the years of working in the fitness industry, I have met many people with health issues ranging from obesity to high cholesterol and high blood pressure to type 2 diabetes. Most of these conditions were a direct result of poor nutritional habits and lack of physical activity. I completed these certifications so I could share my knowledge with others to offer educational information that could assist them to better health. From my experiences and the advice of many doctors, nutritionists and dieticians, I've found that taking charge of nutrition, then adding exercise, is the best combination for success in the weight loss arena. While losing weight, it is also important that individuals take steps to learn what behaviors and habits may have contributed to their medical issues, and how to modify them to support long term sustainability of their newly found health.

I have worked with upwards of 150 people who have followed my nutrition program and they have lost 10, 20, 50 and even 100 pounds, and kept the weight off! It all starts with a decision to get healthy. As a coach, I am there to support and encourage clients, to work on lesson plans for improving behaviors, and to be the sounding board when times get tough. My true joy comes when clients succeed and are able to do the activities they love without restriction from joint pain, lack of energy or taking medications.

My hope is that you will find the tips in this book helpful and educational and that you put some of them into action as you improve your nutrition and physical activity program. You will find resources such as glycemic index tables, a nutrition facts label, BMI chart, and the fat content of meats, poultry and oils on the resource page of my website at ActivationHC.com.

Should you find that you or someone you love could use my guidance to create long term health, please contact me at deenie@activationhc.com.

In health,

Deenie Robertson
Activation Health Coaching

Acknowledgements

This book is dedicated to my Mom, Peggie Reynolds. I am blessed by her love, friendship and unwavering confidence in me. She has a heart of gold and has taught me to be kind, accepting, responsible and reliable, and to never take life too seriously. In addition, I would not be the person I am today without my twins, Evan Robertson and Hayley Schank. I am so very proud of them and their accomplishments, and I love them with all my heart.

I had many friends and family members provide input for this book. I am grateful for the help and encouragement I was given by Jim Peot, the man I love sharing my life with; my mother Peggie Reynolds; my step-father Sherman Reynolds; my daughter-in-law Tiffany Robertson; Tim Cox, Global Director/Certified Health Coach; Jewel Peot, LCSW PhD; and good friends Dr. Stacey Neider, MD and Jolie McGauley. I thank you all, and also give thanks to God for giving me a gift of passion to inspire others to better health.

Forever Healthy Clients of Deenie Robertson

"I wanted you to know that I followed your program and exercise suggestions faithfully for 12 weeks and lost 32 pounds! I had hired a private trainer a year prior to your help and only lost 3 pounds of total weight, gained some muscle, but still was not as lean as I would prefer. I'm six foot, 185 pounds now and my energy levels are very good. My clothes fit me so much better now that it's a pleasure putting on those pants that were too tight before you helped me slim down. I still use your program on a maintenance basis only. I am living proof that the program works when combined with some exercise daily. Recently I had a complete physical and my doctor said my numbers were terrific. Total cholesterol of 134, resting heartbeat of 60, blood pressure of 110/70. He said "Whatever you are doing, keep it up." Oh, by the way, I'll be 59 in October! Thanks for all of your help!" -- *Greg K., Manhattan Beach, California*

"After struggling to lose the weight that had slowly caused my life to go from active to passive, I decided to take serious action to make a change for myself, and for the future. I was "sick and tired of feeling sick and tired"! I knew the extra weight was the problem, and it was time to do something about it. Initially, I was still in denial of the need to lose weight, I felt good enough about myself, it was just that all these "weight-related issues" kept creeping up--pains in my feet, exhaustion

6

most of the time, nausea, just to name a few. When I met Deenie, and decided to commit to making a change, I honestly was relieved and skeptical at the same time. The program and Deenie's support changed all that.

It was like being given a gift beyond measure. The first week on the program I lost 7 pounds, and that was just the beginning! I have slowly and steadily lost weight with Deenie's support and guidance (and with the nutrition program).

To date, 11 months from starting the program, I have lost 52 pounds. My success is better measured in improved attitude, and overall health I have gained. My clothing size dropped from a 16 to a 10. Along the way I have run a triathalon, maintained a weekly swim schedule, changed some unhealthy eating habits and behaviors, and best of all feel younger and happier than I ever have!

Thanks to Deenie for empowering and supporting me through this transformation. I wish you well in your journey to improve your health. I'm looking forward to a bright and healthy future. With Deenie's help you can too!" -- *J. Pepe, Anchorage, Alaska*

"Over the past year, I have lost 40 pounds with the always-supportive help of Deenie! She always makes the call, listens to whatever is on your mind, practices what she teaches and makes me feel like a million bucks even if I don't.

My life has taken a turn for the better with this program, I am no longer diabetic, my blood pressure has lowered, my arthritis went into remission and I have felt so much better about myself. Thanks Deenie for believing in all of us!" -- *M. Miller, Idaho*

"This program is the only program that really helped me to lose weight and keep it off. It is easy to follow and simple. With the help of my online coach Deenie Robertson, who diligently called and e-mailed to see how I was doing. She kept me on track and offered support in times when I needed it.

The program definitely helped me. I feel good inside and out! I have more energy and am eating healthier. I weighed 172 pounds when I started in October 2011 and went down to 143 pounds. I maintained my weight at 145-148. I just started again last month and my goal is to lose 10 more pounds and I have lost 5 already. There is no doubt, the program works!" -- *H. Abiera, Florida*

Table of Contents

Get Your Brain in the Game 11

I'm Too Busy to Eat Healthy 23

Better Nutrition for Fewer Health Risks 35

Which Foods do You Really Need? 47

American Portions are Plumping Us Up 59

How do I Lose Excess Weight? 69

Drink the Calories that Support Health 81

Do I Really Have to Exercise? 93

Snack Times Can be Healthy Times 105

Ten Things to Consider When Shopping 117

Get Your Brain in the Game

1

Get rid of negative self-talk.

Would you tell a friend that she was fat or couldn't achieve a goal? Don't say such things to yourself either! Use positive affirmations such as "I'm getting healthier every day" to build confidence, and notice how attitudes and actions improve!

2

Lack of sleep makes you eat.

Have you ever noticed when you don't get enough sleep you tend to crave sweet or fatty foods? This is your brain playing a trick on you! Adequate sleep (six to eight hours per night) is essential to support good health and nutrition.

3

Diets don't work. Lifestyle changes do.

Many people go on diets to lose weight. Eighty-five percent of them gain the weight back. To be successful when dieting, people must also learn healthier behaviors (like portion control) that will support permanent weight loss.

14

4

Make healthy choices in social situations.

Research shows that we eat more in group settings. If you're meeting your friends for happy hour or a meal, stay away from fried foods, cream sauces and chips, and order a "mocktail" rather than a cocktail.

5

What's most important --health or food?

When you're on your journey to better health and temptations abound, take a moment to remember why your health is important. It will make it easier to say no to foods that will derail your efforts.

6

Support systems can make a difference.

Grab a friend, family member or co-worker to improve her health with you. If you are on a health journey together, you can support and encourage each other and both experience success.

7

Pre-planning menus supports health success.

Choose a day (Sunday works great) to plan your meals for the week. Head to the store with a list to be sure you have all the fruits, veggies, lean protein, whole grains and low-fat dairy that you need.

8

Set health goals, achieve best success.

Why is your health important to you? How will being healthier change your life and activities, and the lives of those around you? Write down your health goals and refer to them often to stay on track for success.

9

Are you hungry or just bored?

Do you ever open the refrigerator door looking for something to eat and realize you're really not hungry? It's common to eat when bored, so next time, drink a glass of water and wait ten minutes before eating.

10

Be mindful, not automatic when eating.

Often we eat quickly without awareness of the foods we're consuming. Slowing down, paying attention to the taste and texture of your food, appreciating the flavors, and putting the fork down between bites can help you eat less.

I'm Too Busy
to Eat Healthy

11

Avoid these foods at all costs.

Fried foods, cream sauces, full-fat creamy salad dressings, whole milk, and high-calorie coffee drinks are all full of fat and calories and can increase your risk for heart disease. Soda is full of sugar and can weaken bones.

12

Eat healthy at the drive-through.

When you have to hit the drive-through, choose a grilled chicken sandwich (only eat half of the bun), or salad with grilled chicken or shrimp. Skip high fat dressings, regular sodas, cheese, bacon and mayo, and don't super-size!

13

Are cheeseburgers really bad for you?

Eating a cheeseburger today will have no effect on your health. Eating a cheeseburger every day will. Red meat should be limited to once a week. Make cheeseburgers at home with lean ground beef, or switch to lean ground turkey.

14

Caesar salad is not your friend.

Don't let the word "salad" trick you into thinking all salads are healthy. Croutons and dressing contain oils and fats that can make your harmless lettuce a 1,000-calorie meal. Order dressing on the side and use sparingly.

15

Good nutrition when you are traveling.

You can make healthy choices when traveling. Ask your server to prepare your order with no added fats, choose lean meats, get dressings on the side, skip the bread basket, and take healthy snacks on the plane with you.

16

But, I don't like to cook.

Stop at the salad bar on the way home. Load up on green, leafy vegetables, beans, mushrooms, and tomatoes, and top with shredded chicken or turkey. Look for low-sodium, low-fat soups in the soup aisle that you can heat and eat.

17

Everyone has a favorite comfort food.

Craving ice cream, mashed potatoes or homemade bread? Switch to low-fat ice cream or sorbet, use skim milk for your potatoes (or mash cauliflower instead), and choose whole-grain bread dipped in a little olive oil.

18

Where are the quick, simple recipes?

Sources abound on the internet for healthy recipes that won't take all night to prepare. Watch for those with reduced fat and sodium, and a close ratio of grams of carbohydrates and lean protein. For recipes and resources, go to ActivationHC.com.

19

Don't derail your diet with condiments.

Condiments like ketchup and barbeque sauce are high in sugar and sodium. Mayonnaise is high in fat. Use condiments sparingly and look for low sugar and low fat versions. Mustard is a great option.

20

Even when busy, don't miss breakfast.

Make some hard boiled eggs to take to work and pair them with a whole-wheat English muffin. Try plain yogurt with fresh fruit or unsweetened cereal with fresh fruit and skim milk. Keep ready-to-eat items on hand for quick breakfasts.

Better Nutrition for Fewer Health Risks

21

Replace white foods with whole grain.

Foods made with refined white flour do nothing for your health (i.e., white bread, sugary cereals, most crackers and chips). Look for varieties made with whole grain to increase your fiber intake and keep you feeling full longer.

22

Best oils to use when cooking

The best oils for cooking are either canola oil or olive oil. Both are low in saturated fat and provide healthy Omega-3s. Olive oil is best used when cooking over low heat, and canola for high heat.

23

Keep blood sugars stabilized all day.

If you feel like you need a nap after eating, it's likely your blood sugar spiked, then dropped due to foods you ate. Eating low-glycemic and high protein meals every two to three hours helps keep blood sugar stable all day.

24

Taking medicine does not create health.

If you've been prescribed medication to manage diabetes, high cholesterol or high blood pressure, know that the medicine alone will not make you healthy. Eating a healthy diet and increasing activity is required to create better health in your life.

25

Live with moderation, variety, and balance.

Choose your foods wisely! It's O.K. to have ice cream or pie, but infrequently and in small portions. Choose a variety of healthy foods--fruits, vegetables, low-fat dairy and lean protein--to eat 90 percent of the time.

26

Cardiovascular disease comes from lifestyle choices.

Cardiovascular (heart) disease can be prevented by reducing intake of high-fat foods and incorporating more exercise. Shop for more whole foods like oatmeal, fruits and vegetables, and avoid packaged foods, especially if they contain trans fats.

41

27

Type 2 diabetes can be prevented.

Most people with type 2 diabetes are diagnosed with the disease due to poor food choices and lack of exercise. If it runs in your family, don't wait to start improving your nutrition and physical activity to reduce your risk.

28

Fat is often replaced with sugar.

When a food product says "fat-free," generally the manufacturer has added sugar to make up for the reduction in fat. While you may consume less fat, you will get more sugar, which is not necessarily a good trade-off.

29

Yes, stress can create nutritional deficiencies.

Stress can result in cravings for foods high in fat, sugar and salt. Stress causes increased cortisol production which can lead to weight gain and depletion of B vitamins, vitamin C, zinc and magnesium. Stress management improves your health!

30

How do you eat an antioxidant?

Antioxidants may reduce risk for heart disease or cancer. Shop for fruits high in vitamin C like kiwi, oranges, papaya, guava and strawberries, and vegetables such as spinach, broccoli, brussels sprouts, kale, cauliflower, red chili and bell peppers.

Which Foods do You Really Need?

31

Which food groups are the healthiest?

Fruits, vegetables, lean protein (chicken, turkey, fish), low-fat dairy (skim milk, low-fat yogurt, reduced fat cheese), and whole grains (oatmeal, bran, whole wheat) provide the essential nutrients our bodies need to function and stave off disease.

32

Which foods keep you feeling full?

Choosing foods that contain protein (lean meat, tofu, and eggs) and high fiber (beans, green leafy vegetables and whole grain breads and cereals) will help you stay full longer, which can contribute to eating less and staying healthy.

33

How much protein do you need?

Most of us get plenty of protein every day without even trying. If you are eating low-fat dairy and lean protein like chicken, fish, tofu or even eggs, you will easily meet your daily requirements.

34

Is "sugar-free" better for you?

Sugar-free products reduce calories, but consume them in moderation. Artificial sweeteners go through chemical processes before they get to you. Some products have been linked to increased risk of cancer. They also entice your brain to want more sugar.

35

Are carbohydrates really bad for you?

If you think of bread, rice, or pasta when you hear "carbohydrates," consider switching to whole grain varieties to improve their nutritional value. Don't forget carbs are also present in fruit and vegetables. So, not all carbs are bad.

36

Your favorite veggie could be unhealthy.

Potatoes and onions are healthy. French fries and blooming onions are not! You are not contributing to good health if your veggie is fried or smothered in butter. Switch to a sweet potato, and sauté your onions with green veggies.

37

Bodies need fiber. Get it here.

Bodies need both soluble (absorbs water) and insoluble fiber to maintain regularity and bowel health. Get soluble fiber in oatmeal, barley, beans and citrus fruits; and get insoluble fiber in fruits like apple with peel, vegetables, and whole grain breads and cereals.

38

Quinoa, wild rice and sweet potatoes.

These low-glycemic foods help control blood sugar and reduce the spike of insulin levels. All vegetables, fruits, legumes, starchy and sugary foods have glycemic ratings. Low-glycemic, whole grain starches are critical for good health.

39

Best choices in the fruit aisle

Fruit is good for you. Period. Choosing low-glycemic fruits can be even better if you're trying to control blood sugar or lose weight. Your best low-glycemic choices are berries and citrus fruits, apples, nectarines, plums, peaches and pears.

40

What's the problem with eating fat?

We need fat in our diets, but often it's high in saturated and trans fats which increase risks of heart disease. Choose healthy fats in foods like salmon, olive oil, nuts, avocados, and low-fat dairy. Be sure to measure portion sizes.

American Portions are Plumping Us Up

41

Eat plenty, but don't super-size.

Don't fall prey to the temptation to "super-size" your meals! The extra food increases your calorie, fat, sodium and carbohydrate intake. Large portions eaten in restaurants or at home may be a major contributing factor to weight gain.

42

Always use a nine-inch plate.

Standard dinner plates are about twelve inches. By switching to a nine-inch plate, you will reduce portion sizes and calorie intake. Cover 50 percent of the plate with fruits and vegetables, 25 percent with low-glycemic starches and 25 percent with lean protein.

43

Two decks of cards for dinner

One serving of lean protein is about the size of a deck of cards, or three ounces. Most people should be eating a six-ounce portion of lean protein at a dinner meal--the equivalent of two decks of cards.

44

How to eat a tennis ball

Most everyone seems to love starchy foods-- potatoes, rice, pasta and bread. Keep your portions to the size of a tennis ball or about one half-cup and choose whole grain and lower-glycemic starches like quinoa when- ever you can.

45

Roll the dice
when eating cheese.

Cheese--such a wonderful food to enjoy! Unfortunately it is also filled with fat. Choose reduced-fat cheeses and keep portion sizes to one ounce—about the size of four dice. Choose full-fat cheeses for special occasions only.

46

What does "moderation" really mean anyway?

Moderation means not too much or too little of anything. It doesn't mean you have to eliminate high fat foods or sugar, but that you have them occasionally in small amounts. In other words, don't take things to extremes.

47

Today's muffins contribute to muffin tops.

How could you go wrong with blueberry or bran muffins? Today's muffins are easily double the size they were in the 1960s, and instead of 100 calories each, they can pack as many as 500, with upwards of 30 grams of fat!

48

Bagels and popcorn have plumped up!

Bagels have grown from a mere three-inch diameter to between five and six inches. Movie popcorn servings used to be about five cups and are now a huge tub. Stick with half of a bagel, and skip the butter flavored movie popcorn!

49

Twice a month equals two pounds.

Two slices of pepperoni pizza have 350 more calories today than in the 1980s. Two slices, twice a month, can add up to two extra pounds a year! Try a veggie pizza on whole wheat crust instead.

How do I Lose Excess Weight?

50

What are you having for breakfast?

You've probably heard it before, but breakfast is the most important meal of the day! Studies show that people who eat breakfast eat fewer calories by the end of the day. Choose a breakfast with a balance of carbohydrate and lean protein like whole wheat toast and poached eggs.

51

You don't need the whole bun.

If you love burgers--even if they're chicken or turkey burgers--you can save yourself calories by eating only half of the bun, or lose the bun completely (especially if it is made of white enriched flour).

52

Eating fiber can keep you thin.

When you eat foods with fiber such as oranges, apples, and whole grains, your body has to work harder to digest them. Not only do you get more nutrients when you eat high fiber foods, but your body will burn more calories!

53

Which is better?
Skinny or healthy?

You may look at someone who is "skinny" and think he or she is healthy but that may not be the case. Is that person getting proper nutrients? Are they maintaining muscle mass? Healthy means eating properly and getting regular activity.

54

Eating like kings, princes and paupers

There's a saying out there, "Eat breakfast like a king, lunch like a prince, and dinner like a pauper." Studies show that eating your big meal earlier in the day (breakfast or lunch) contributes to greater weight loss.

55

How many calories do I need?

To maintain your weight, multiply your current weight by 11. That number equals the calories you need to consume if you are sedentary. Reduce that number by 500 to lose weight. Increase by 1.2 if you get moderate exercise.

56

Timing of meals makes a difference.

Fueling your body regularly throughout the day will keep your metabolism burning hot. Have your first meal within one hour of waking, and then eat small, low-fat meals every two to three hours the rest of the day.

57

Reduce added sugars in your diet.

To reduce sugars you consume, use fewer added sugars like white or brown sugar, honey and syrups. Limit soft drinks, candy, ice cream and high-sugar cereals. Read nutrition labels to monitor the sugars included in processed foods.

58

I'm too busy to count calories.

Take time to calculate the calories in your favorite foods and write them down. Then plan for a 300 to 500-calorie breakfast, lunch and dinner, and three 100-calorie snacks. Modify total calories for your weight goal.

59

Will cutting gluten help weight loss?

Many people choose gluten-free diets even if they don't really have the need. There has been no evidence that eating a gluten-free diet will assist in losing weight. Skip this fad diet if you don't have a gluten intolerance or allergy.

Drink the Calories that Support Health

60

Caffeine--it's not just in coffee.

When we hear "caffeine" we immediately think coffee, but it's also in tea, soft drinks, energy drinks and chocolate. Limit caffeine to 200 to 300 milligrams per day, which is two to four cups of brewed coffee.

61

Your coffee drink makes a difference.

A cup of coffee has zero calories. Add two tablespoons of "half-and-half" and it becomes 40 calories with three grams of fat. A 16-ounce nonfat Caramel Macchiato has 240 calories, one gram of fat and 32 grams of sugar. Check nutrition facts before ordering!

62

Water, water, water. Drink it up!

Water makes up 45 to 75 percent of our body weight, and is absolutely essential to life. Water moves nutrients and waste between cells and organs, carries food through your digestive system, and regulates your heating/cooling system.

63

Whole fruit's better than fruit juice.

Fruit juices are fine to drink once in a while, but whole fruit is better. Read labels on juices. Look for 100 percent fruit juice and check the calorie counts and grams of sugar. Some have more sugar than a soda!

64

Are there benefits to drinking alcohol?

Some experts believe so, but not for everyone. Compared with people who rarely drink, those who drink slightly have shown lower mortality rates. The benefit is seen in those who consume one drink per *week*.

65

Are there negatives to drinking alcohol?

Alcohol has calories but is not a nutrient. It interferes with normal nutrition by affecting absorption, metabolism and excretion of many vitamins and minerals. Alcohol increases fluid loss. Excessive alcohol consumption deprives the brain of oxygen and stresses the liver.

66

Ten teaspoons of sugar for lunch

Would you eat ten sugar cubes for lunch? If you have a regular 12-ounce soda, that's exactly what you're doing! That's 150 calories of pure sugar and an increased risk for diabetes. One daily soda equals 15.64 pounds gained per year.

67

Energize your morning the healthy way.

Start your day by drinking an eight-ounce glass of water. It will replace the fluids you lost while sleeping, give you a burst of energy, and offset dehydration that starts with your first caffeinated beverage of the day.

68

Not all fruit smoothies are healthy.

Some chain store smoothies are more than 300 calories, full of sugar and carbo-hydrates, and low on protein. Make yours at home with protein powder, water and frozen fruit. Add a scoop of ground flaxseed for an extra health benefit.

69

If you're thirsty, it's too late.

Thirst is not always a reliable guide to when you should drink. By the time dehydration triggers the thirst stimulus, you will have lost one to two percent of your body weight in water. Keep a water bottle handy all day.

Do I Really Have to Exercise?

70

Which exercise helps me get healthy?

Cardiovascular exercise, such as walking, swimming, bicycling and running, increase the heart rate, burn calories and reduce the risk of chronic disease. Exercises like lifting weights or yoga increase strength, flexibility and endurance which help maintain muscle mass as we age.

71

How much exercise is recommended now?

The general recommendation is moderate intensity cardiovascular activity at least 30 minutes per day, six days per week. If you're just starting, begin slowly and increase the time and intensity each week. Get clearance from your doctor first.

72

Will sit-ups make my stomach flat?

Sit-ups and other core exercises are a great way to improve abdominal strength. If done correctly, they can contribute to a flatter stomach. If you carry weight around your waist, reduce the fat to show off your strong tummy!

73

Exercise doesn't have to be painful.

If you hear the word exercise and immediately panic, know that what is most important is moving your body (physical activity). The most efficient activity to improve your health is walking. Start slowly, and then increase the distance and intensity.

74

Burn calories while you're at work.

Simple things you do daily can burn more calories if done with purpose. Focus on sitting up straight in meetings and get up often. Stand when you're on the phone. Conduct meetings while walking. Walk during your lunch hour.

75

Take a step back to childhood.

What activities did you love as a kid? Riding your bike, jumping rope, climbing trees? Chances are you would still like doing those activities now. Finding activities you love will help you stick with a physical activity program.

76

What's the best time to exercise?

Research shows that exercise first thing in the morning can be the most effective, mostly because it's easier to add to your schedule before your day becomes busy. Your best time will be when you can do it consistently.

77

What are the benefits of exercise?

Exercise can increase energy, reduce stress, help you sleep better, improve self-confidence, and help maintain a healthy weight. It can also prevent osteoporosis and cardiovascular disease, get you outside, and help prevent chronic disease. Find something you enjoy, and do it!

78

Adding exercise to a busy schedule

Start your day by waking up 10 to 30 minutes earlier and walk, stretch or do core work. If you prefer to work out later, schedule it on your calendar like an important work meeting and don't be late!

79

Fidgeting can help burn more calories.

Toe tapping, playing guitar, singing, chewing gum and fidgeting can all contribute to your daily calorie burn by up to 20 percent! Movement is a key piece of losing and maintaining weight even if it doesn't seem like much.

Snack Times Can be Healthy Times

80

Healthy snacking while out and about

Need a quick snack but your only choice is a local convenience store or fast food establishment? Choose fresh fruit, nonfat yogurt, three ounces of non-fat frozen yogurt or no more than one and a half ounces of mixed nuts.

81

Nighttime snacks-- the do's and don'ts

The key to nighttime snacks is to make them small, low-fat and low-calorie. Pop your own popcorn in the microwave in a covered dish with a little water. Three cups has only 90 calories.

82

Kick the craving for afternoon sweets.

Reducing sugars throughout the day can reduce sweet cravings. Snack on a fresh peach or nonfat yogurt with berries. One square of dark chocolate with 70 percent or higher cacao content and five almonds makes a great blood-pressure-reducing treat.

83

Is it too late to eat?

If you've followed a healthy eating plan during the day--three portion controlled main meals and two healthy snacks--there is nothing wrong with having another healthy snack before bed. Keep it to 100 low-fat calories or less.

84

Do nuts make a healthy snack?

Nuts are a great healthy snack, but watch portion sizes. While nuts provide protein and healthy fats, they are high in calories. A healthy portion of nuts is about 1.5 ounces equaling 24 almonds, 28 peanuts or 14 walnut halves.

85

It's easy getting five a day.

It is recommended to eat five servings of fruits and/or vegetables per day. Add these nutritious snacks to your day: one orange, pear or apple; one cup of cherries; two cups of raspberries; one-half cup of sliced cucumbers; half an avocado; or two cups of baby carrots.

86

Get your veggies and dip 'em!

Snack time can be a great time to increase your veggie intake for the day. Choose a half-cup cucumber slices, six celery sticks, or a half-cup raw broccoli florets and dip in two ounces of low-fat or sugar-free dressing.

87

Beware the bagel with cream cheese.

Today's bagels are oversized and high in calories. If you're craving that bread-like carb, try a slice of whole grain bread with two ounces of fat-free turkey breast or a tablespoon of reduced fat cream cheese.

88

Warm your belly to stay full.

Eating a warm bowl of soup can help you feel full without a lot of calories. Try a cup of chicken noodle, vegetable or reduced-fat cream of tomato to get you through afternoon hunger pangs.

89

Beans are another great snack option.

Try one cup of bean and chickpea salad, one-fourth cup of hummus with celery or tomato, one-half cup edamame (soybeans), or one cup of vegetarian chili to add fiber and protein to your diet.

Ten Things to Consider When Shopping

90

The middle aisles expand your waistline.

Did you ever notice that fruits and vegetables are on one side of the store, with dairy and meats on the other? Stick to the outside perimeter for the healthiest foods. The middle aisles are full of processed, unhealthy options.

91

Farmers markets are a nutrition goldmine.

Farmers markets provide you with locally grown foods at the peak of growing season, rather than produce that's been picked weeks before arriving at the grocery store. Fresher fruits and veggies provide more vitamins, antioxidants and phytochemicals.

92

The important information on nutrition labels.

Most people focus on calories, grams, or milligrams. But "Percent Daily Value" on packages breaks down the nutritional value of your product. Percent Daily Value under 5 percent is low, 20 percent is high. Choose values low in fat, cholesterol and sodium; high in fiber, vitamins and minerals.

93

Fill cart with freshness, not packages.

It's hard to avoid all packaged foods, but use common sense when you shop. Shop for fresh vegetables and fruits, local meats, fresh or recently frozen fish and skip the packaged cookies, chips, high-sugar cereals and frozen meals.

94

Which foods should
I buy organic?

Buying organic means you consume fewer pesticides. Consider purchasing apples, celery and strawberries that are organic. According to foodnews.org, peaches, spinach, nectarines, grapes and sweet bell peppers are best purchased organic. Always wash produce before eating or cooking.

95

Don't go shopping when you're hungry.

Have a snack before you head to the grocery store to reduce the chances of impulse purchases, and purchasing foods that are not healthy (but tempting!). If your store is offering free food samples, stick with tasting the healthy ones.

96

There is a difference in waters.

Distilled and purified waters may have removed chemicals and contaminants, but in the process lose natural minerals. Spring water may or may not have been treated. Tap water may be your best choice, but check with your local EPA.

97

Use a basket,
not a cart.

If you've got to make a quick run to the store after work, pick up a small hand-carried basket rather than a cart to reduce purchasing unnecessary or unhealthy items. Stick to your list and you'll save calories and money!

98

Don't leave home without a list!

Do your best to grocery shop one day a week, and be sure to have your list with you. Not only will this help with meal planning, but it will save calories, time, extra trips to the store, and money.

99

Buy functional foods for health benefits.

Functional foods provide health benefits beyond basic nutrition. Garlic, and fiber from oatmeal may reduce heart disease risk. Tomato sauce may reduce prostate cancer risk. Phytochemicals (pigments and antioxidants) from plants protect from heart disease, hypertension, cancer and diabetes.

100

Identify fraudulent products when you shop.

Watch for claims made in labeling and advertising. Be wary of products stating a secret cure, breakthrough, or new discovery. Be careful of items that detoxify, purify or energize, and those with scientific studies but no list of references. If the claims were true, health professionals would know!

Presentations by Activation Health Coaching

Deenie Robertson is the owner of Activation Health Coaching and has done presentations for a variety of businesses interested in learning about the benefits of employee wellness programs, and educating their employees on the benefits of better nutrition, improved sleep, and stress management.

Whether your company has an established wellness program or not, Deenie is an accomplished speaker who brings easy-to-use tips into the workplace so employees can immediately start putting the information into action.

Deenie has done presentations, both in person and via web-conferencing, for chambers of commerce, insurance brokers, and other large corporations in both Alaska and Washington.

To reserve a presentation for your next wellness event, please contact Deenie at deenie@activationhc.com or at ActivationHC.com.

See the entire Six-Word Lesson Series at
6wordlessons.com

Want to learn more about being
healthy forever?

Contact Deenie at
ActivationHC.com

Read more about Deenie at
ActivationHC.com